Table of Contents

Alzheimer's disease is a progressive neurologic disorder that causes the brain to shrink (atrophy) and brain cells to die. Alzheimer's disease is the most common cause of dementia — a continuous decline in thinking, behavioral and social skills that affects a person's ability to function independently.

Approximately 5.8 million people in the United States age 65 and older live with Alzheimer's disease. Of those, 80% are 75 years old and older. Out of the approximately 50 million people worldwide with dementia, between 60% and 70% are estimated to have Alzheimer's disease.

The early signs of the disease include forgetting recent events or conversations. As the disease progresses, a person with Alzheimer's disease will develop severe memory impairment and lose the ability to carry out everyday tasks.

Medications may temporarily improve or slow progression of symptoms. These treatments can sometimes help people with Alzheimer's disease maximize function and maintain independence for a time. Different programs and services can help support people with Alzheimer's disease and their caregivers.

There is no treatment that cures Alzheimer's disease or alters the disease process in the brain. In advanced stages of the disease, complications from severe loss of brain function — such as dehydration, malnutrition or infection — result in death.

BREAKFAST

1. Breakfast Pizza

Prep Time: 10 Minutes

Cook Time: 20 Minutes

Servings: 6

Ingredients

- 1 pkg. Crescent Rolls
- 8 ounces Jimmy Dean Sausage – (regular, hot or maple) (you can use more or less to taste)
- 1 cup Shredded Hash Browns – thawed
- 1 cup Shredded Cheese – Mexican Blend or your favorite cheese.
- 5 eggs
- 1/4 cup milk
- 1/2 teaspoon salt
- 1/2 teaspoon pepper
- 2 tablespoon Parmesan – grated

Equipment

- Baking Sheet

Instructions

1. Preheat oven to 375 degrees.

2. Take the Crescent Rolls out of the fridge 15 minutes before making.
3. Spray small sheet pan (10×15) with nonstick spray. (For a deeper style pizza, you can make in a 9×13 casserole dish!)
4. Brown the sausage in a skillet and drain.
5. Spread the rolls on prepared pan.
6. You will have to press and work the dough a little to make sure it covers the pan...pinch the pieces together.
7. Spoon sausage over the crust.
8. Spread the potatoes over the meat.
9. Spread the cheese over the potatoes.
10. Combine eggs, milk, salt, pepper, parmesan together in a separate bowl.
11. Spoon the egg mixture evenly over the cheese.
12. (TO RECAP THE LAYERING: ROLLS, MEAT, POTATOES, CHEESE, EGG MIXTURE)
13. Bake at 375 degrees for 25-30 minutes or until eggs are set. Oven times vary so check it about half way through.

Prep Time: 10 Minutes

Cook Time: 30 Minutes

Servings: 12

Ingredients

- ½ cup unsalted butter 113 grams, melted (1 stick)
- 1 cup granulated sugar 200 grams
- 2 large eggs 100 grams, room temperature
- 3 bananas mashed
- ¾ cup buttermilk 170 grams, room temperature
- 2 teaspoons pure vanilla extracts 8 grams
- 2 cups all-purpose flour 240 grams
- 2 teaspoons baking powder 8 grams
- 1 teaspoon baking soda 6 grams
- 1 teaspoon kosher salt 3 grams
- 1½ cups mini chocolate chips 266 grams, divided

Equipment

- Kitchen Scale (optional)
- 9×13 Baking Pan
- Hand Mixer (optional)

Instructions

1. Preheat oven to 350°F. Grease a 9×13-inch baking pan with nonstick spray. Set aside.

2. In a large bowl, with a whisk or hand mixer, beat the butter, sugar, and eggs together.
3. ½ cup unsalted butter,1 cup granulated sugar,2 large eggs
4. Add the banana, buttermilk, and vanilla and mix well.
5. 3 bananas,¾ cup buttermilk,2 teaspoons pure vanilla extract
6. Stir in the flour, baking powder, baking soda, and salt.
7. 2 cups all-purpose flour,2 teaspoons baking powder,1 teaspoon baking soda,1 teaspoon salt
8. Fold in 1¼ cups of the chocolate chips.
9. 1½ cups mini chocolate chips
10. Pour the batter into the prepared pan.
11. Sprinkle the remaining chocolate chips over the top.
12. Bake for 30 minutes, or until a toothpick comes out clean.
13. Allow to cool completely in the pan before cutting into squares.

Prep Time: 10 Minutes

Cook Time: 1hrs 10 Minutes

Servings: 13

Ingredients

- 1½ cups shelled pistachios 180 grams
- 1½ cups Honey Roasted Almond Slices 129 grams, Fresh Gourmet recommended
- 1 cup rolled oats 100 grams
- 1 cup roasted pepitas (pumpkin seeds) 119 grams
- ½ cup steel-cut oats 99 grams
- 1 teaspoon kosher salt 3 grams
- ½ cup brown sugar 107 grams
- ⅓ cup pure maple syrup 104 grams
- ⅓ cup canola oil 67 grams
- ½ cup dried blueberries 85 grams
- ½ cup dried cranberries 85 grams

Equipment

- Kitchen Scale (optional)
- Baking Sheet

Instructions

1. Preheat oven to 350°F and line a large baking sheet with aluminum foil. Spray the foil with nonstick cooking spray.
2. In a large mixing bowl, mix together all granola ingredients except the blueberries and cranberries.

3. 1½ cups shelled pistachios,1½ cups Honey Roasted Almond Slices,1 cup rolled oats,1 cup roasted pepitas (pumpkin seeds),½ cup steel-cut oats,1 teaspoon kosher salt,½ cup brown sugar,⅓ cup pure maple syrup,⅓ cup canola oil
4. Spread the granola ingredients evenly onto the prepared baking sheet and bake for 40 minutes, stirring halfway through. Granola should be golden brown and crunchy.
5. Remove from the oven and stir in the dried blueberries and cranberries (SEE NOTE).
6. ½ cup dried blueberries,½ cup dried cranberries
7. Cool completely before enjoying.

Prep Time: 10 Minutes

Cook Time: 20 Minutes

Servings: 12

Ingredients

- ⅓ cup vegetable oil 67 grams
- 1 cup granulated sugar 200 grams
- ½ cup sour cream 114 grams
- ½ cup buttermilk 114 grams
- 1 large egg 50 grams
- 1 teaspoon pure vanilla extracts 4 grams
- 1½ cups all-purpose flour 180 grams, plus 2 teaspoons (5 grams) for the blueberries
- ½ teaspoon kosher salt
- 2 teaspoons baking powder 8 grams
- 1½ cups fresh blueberries 255 grams
- Brown Sugar Topping
- ½ cup brown sugar 107 grams
- ¼ cup all-purpose flour 30 grams
- 2 tablespoons unsalted butter 28 grams, melted (¼ stick)

Equipment

- Kitchen Scale (optional)
- Muffin Tin

Instructions

1. Preheat oven to 375°F. Grease a 12-count muffin tin or line with paper liners. Set aside.
2. Whisk together oil and sugar until fluffy.
3. ⅓ cup vegetable oil,1 cup granulated sugar
4. Whisk in sour cream, buttermilk, egg, and vanilla until just combined.
5. ½ cup sour cream,½ cup buttermilk,1 large egg,1 teaspoon pure vanilla extract
6. Add in 1½ cups flour, salt, and baking powder and stir. Do not overmix.
7. 1½ cups all-purpose flour,½ teaspoon kosher salt,2 teaspoons baking powder
8. Toss fresh blueberries with 2 teaspoons of flour until all the blueberries are coated.
9. 1½ cups fresh blueberries
10. Add the blueberries into the mixture and gently fold until incorporated, making sure not to break any of the berries.
11. Spoon blueberry mixture into the prepared muffin tin until each well is ⅔ full.
12. Prepare brown sugar topping by stirring together brown sugar, flour, and melted butter.
13. ½ cup brown sugar,¼ cup all-purpose flour,2 tablespoons unsalted butter
14. Sprinkle each muffin with a generous coating of brown sugar topping.
15. Bake in oven for 20 to 25 minutes, or until muffins spring back when touched or toothpick comes out clean.
16. Let muffins cool on a wire rack.

Prep Time: 10 Minutes

Cook Time: 20 Minutes

Servings: 4

Ingredients

- 4 tablespoons unsalted butter for spreading (½ stick)
- 4 English muffins halved
- 8 slices Canadian bacon
- 8 large eggs
- 1 tablespoon white vinegar

For the Hollandaise

- 4 tablespoons unsalted butter ½ stick
- 1 tablespoon lemon juice from ½ lemon
- 1 teaspoon Dijon mustard
- 4 egg yolks

For Serving

- Salt and pepper optional, to taste
- Chopped fresh chives optional
- Ground paprika optional

Equipment

- Baking Sheet
- High Powered Blender Optional
- Food Processor Optional

Instructions

1. Butter the English muffin halves and place them on a baking sheet, cut side up.
2. 4 tablespoons unsalted butter,4 English muffins
3. Add the Canadian bacon to the same baking sheet.
4. 8 slices Canadian bacon
5. Place the sheet under the broiler for 3-4 minutes until the English muffins are toasted and the Canadian bacon is crisped on the edges.
6. In a large saucepan, bring water to a boil.
7. Crack the eggs into small bowls or ramekins.
8. 8 large eggs
9. Reduce the heat so the water is barely simmering with just a few tiny bubbles at the bottom of the pan.
10. Add 1 tablespoon of vinegar to the water.
11. 1 tablespoon white vinegar
12. Bring the ramekins close to the water and gently drop in the eggs, 2-4 at a time.
13. Cover the pan, letting the eggs poach for about 4 minutes.
14. Use a slotted spoon to transfer the eggs to a plate lined with paper towel. Set aside.

For the Hollandaise Sauce:

1. Melt the butter in the microwave.
2. 4 tablespoons unsalted butter
3. Add the lemon juice, Dijon mustard, and egg yolks to a blender or food processor and blend until smooth, about 1 minute.
4. 1 tablespoon lemon juice,1 teaspoon Dijon mustard,4 egg yolks
5. Keeping the blender running, slowly stream in the melted butter.

6. Blend until the mixture reaches a smooth and slightly thickened consistency.
7. Assembly
8. Place one slice of Canadian bacon on each English muffin half. Then, top with a poached egg.
9. Spoon Hollandaise sauce over each egg.
10. Finish with a sprinkle of salt and pepper, chives, and paprika, if desired.
11. Salt and pepper,Chopped fresh chives,Ground paprika

Prep Time: 15 Minutes

Cook Time: 30 Minutes

Servings: 4

Ingredients

- 4 tablespoons unsalted butter room temperature and divided (½ stick)
- 4 large eggs
- ⅛ teaspoon salt
- ⅛ teaspoon ground black pepper
- 4 croissants cut in half lengthwise
- 12 slices thin-sliced deli ham
- 4 slices baby swiss cheese

Equipment

- Baking Sheet

Instructions

1. Preheat oven to 350°F and line a baking sheet with parchment paper. Set aside.
2. overhead view of ingredients for croissant breakfast sandwiches.
3. Heat 1 tablespoon of the butter in a skillet set over medium heat. Add the eggs and whisk until they are cooked through.
4. 4 tablespoons unsalted butter,4 large eggs
5. scrambled eggs in a frying pan.
6. Stir in the salt and pepper then remove from the heat.

7. ⅛ teaspoon kosher salt,⅛ teaspoon ground black pepper
8. Spread some butter on each side of the croissants then fold 3 slices of ham and place them on the bottom side of the croissant.
9. 4 croissants,12 slices thin-sliced deli ham
10. 4 slices of ham on a buttered half croissant on a white plate.
11. Add some eggs on top then spread it out and add a piece of cheese then top it off with the top half of the croissant.
12. 4 slices baby swiss cheese
13. cheese on top of eggs and ham on a buttered half croissant.
14. Place the sandwich on the baking tray then make the rest of the sandwiches and bake for 15 minutes.
15. 4 croissant breakfast sandwiches on a baking sheet.
16. Let the sandwiches cool for 3-4 minutes before serving.

Prep Time: 15 Minutes

Cook Time: 10 Minutes

Servings: 4

Ingredients

- 1 cup cubed red potatoes
- 1 cup cubed white potatoes
- 1 tablespoon olive oil
- ½ teaspoon dried thyme
- ½ teaspoon ground black pepper
- 2 tablespoons salted butter
- 1 white onion diced
- 2 cups cubed fresh corned beef about ¼ pound
- Chopped fresh parsley for garnish

Instructions

1. Preheat oven to 400°F. Line a baking sheet with parchment paper or spray a baking sheet with nonstick spray. Set aside.
2. ingredients for corned beef hash
3. In a medium bowl combine the potatoes, oil, thyme, and pepper. Mix until the potatoes are evenly coated.
4. 1 cup cubed red potatoes,1 cup cubed white potatoes,1 tablespoon olive oil,½ teaspoon dried thyme,½ teaspoon ground black pepper
5. seasoned diced potatoes in a glass bowl
6. Pour the potatoes onto the prepared baking sheet. Spread them into an even layer.

7. diced potatoes on a baking sheet
8. Bake the potatoes for 20 minutes, until golden brown.
9. While the potatoes cook, melt the butter in a cast iron skillet set over medium-high heat. Add the onions and cook for 2-3 minutes.
10. 2 tablespoons salted butter,1 white onion
11. diced onion in a skillet
12. Add the corned beef to the skillet and cook for another 4-5 minutes.
13. 2 cups cubed fresh corned beef
14. diced onion and corned beef in a skillet
15. When the potatoes are golden brown, remove them from the oven and add to the skillet. Mix well and cook for 2-3 minutes. Serve with parsley and enjoy.
16. Chopped fresh parsley
17. potatoes and corned beef in a skillet.

Prep Time: 15 Minutes

Cook Time: 40 Minutes

Servings: 8

Ingredients

- 2¼ cups old-fashioned oats 225 grams
- ½ cup brown sugar 107 grams
- 1 teaspoon baking powder 4 grams
- ¼ teaspoon allspice
- 2 cups half-and-half 454 grams, room temperature
- 2 large eggs 100 grams, room temperature
- 2 tablespoons salted butter 28 grams, melted (¼ stick)
- 1 tablespoon lemon juice 14 grams, from ½ lemon
- 1 tablespoon honey 22 grams
- ½ teaspoon pure vanilla extract 2 grams
- 2 cups blueberries 340 grams
- 1 cup chopped pecans 114 grams

For Serving (optional)

- Honey
- Maple syrup
- Fresh Fruit
- Yogurt

Equipment

- Kitchen Scale (optional)
- 8×8-inch Baking Pan

Instructions

1. Preheat oven to 375°F. Spray an 8×8-inch baking pan with nonstick spray. Set aside.
2. ingredients for blueberry baked oatmeal
3. In a large bowl, whisk the oats, brown sugar, baking powder, and allspice together.
4. 2¼ cups old-fashioned oats,½ cup brown sugar,1 teaspoon baking powder,¼ teaspoon allspice
5. dry ingredients for blueberry baked oatmeal
6. In another bowl, mix the half-and-half, eggs, butter, lemon juice, honey, and vanilla extract together until well combined.
7. 2 cups half-and-half,2 large eggs,2 tablespoons salted butter,1 tablespoon lemon juice,1 tablespoon honey,½ teaspoon pure vanilla extract
8. ingredients for blueberry baked oatmeal
9. Pour the milk mixture into the oats. Mix well.
10. oatmeal mixture in a glass bowl with a wood spoon
11. Gently fold in the blueberries and pecans.
12. 2 cups blueberries,1 cup chopped pecans
13. adding nuts and blueberries to oatmeal mixture in a glass bowl
14. Transfer the batter into the prepared baking pan and spread it into an even layer.
15. blueberry baked oatmeal before baking
16. Bake for 40-45 minutes or until golden brown. Let cool before plating and serving.
17. Honey

Prep Time: 15 Minutes

Cook Time: 1hrs 40 Minutes

Servings: 18

Ingredients

- 2 cups all-purpose flour 240 grams
- 1 teaspoon baking soda 6 grams
- ½ teaspoon baking powder 2 grams
- ½ teaspoon salt
- ½ cup unsalted butter 113 grams, melted (1 stick)
- 6 ripe bananas mashed (about 3 cups or 675 grams)
- ½ cup brown sugar 107 grams
- ¼ cup granulated sugar 50 grams
- 2 large eggs 100 grams, room temperature
- 1 teaspoon pure vanilla extract 4 grams
- ⅓ cup Nutella 90 grams, store-bought or homemade

Equipment

- Kitchen Scale (optional)
- 2 Muffin Tin
- Hand Mixer

Instructions

1. Preheat oven to 350°F. Line two 12-count muffin tins with 18 paper liners. Set aside.
2. overhead view of ingredients for banana nutella muffins.

3. In a medium bowl, whisk the flour, baking soda, baking powder, and salt together. Set aside.

4. 2 cups all-purpose flour,1 teaspoon baking soda,½ teaspoon baking powder,½ teaspoon kosher salt

5. dry ingredients for banana nutella muffins in a glass bowl next to a half-dozen eggs, a peeled banana, and nutella.

6. Using a hand mixer, beat the butter, bananas, brown sugar, sugar, eggs, and vanilla together on medium speed for 3 minutes. Gently stir in the flour mixture until just combined. Set aside.

7. ½ cup unsalted butter,6 ripe bananas,½ cup brown sugar,¼ cup granulated sugar,2 large eggs,1 teaspoon pure vanilla extract

8. banana nutella muffin batter in a glass bowl next to a half-dozen eggs, a peeled banana, and nutella.

9. Place the Nutella in a small microwave-safe bowl and warm for 30 seconds until it's thinned.

10. ⅓ cup Nutella

11. Fill the wells of the muffin tins so they are ¾ full. Spoon the Nutella over the batter, and swirl them together with a knife.

12. nutella swirled into banana muffin batter in a muffin tin.

13. Bake for 15-18 minutes, until a toothpick is inserted in the center of the loaf and it comes out clean.

14. baked banana nutella muffins in a muffin tin.

15. Move the muffins over to a cooling rack and allow them to cool for 15 minutes.

10. Cheesy Sausage and Potatoes

Prep Time: 10 Minutes

Cook Time: 20 Minutes

Servings: 8

Ingredients

- 3 pounds Yukon Gold potatoes peeled and cut into ¼-inch slices
- ¼ cup unsalted butter melted
- 1 pound bulk hot pork sausage
- 1 medium yellow onion chopped
- 2 cups shredded cheese; cheddar Gruyere, Swiss or a mixture
- 2 tablespoons chopped fresh parsley for garnish

Instructions

1. Heat oven to 350°F and spray 13x9-inch baking dish with nonstick cooking spray.
2. Place potatoes in a large saucepan, over medium-high heat, and cover them with cold water. Bring the water to a boil and reduce the heat to low. Cook, uncovered 8-10 minutes or until the potatoes are just fork tender. Drain the potatoes and place them in the prepared baking dish.
3. Pour the melted butter over the potatoes.
4. While the potatoes cook, crumble the sausage in a large skillet set over medium heat. Add the chopped onion and cook until the onion is translucent and the sausage is cooked through. Transfer the

sausage/onion mixture to a paper towel-lined plate
and dab the top of the mixture with another paper
towel.
5. Spread the sausage/onion mixture over the potatoes
and gently toss the mixture together.
6. Top with cheese and bake, uncovered, at 350°F for 7-
10 minutes or until the cheese is melted.
7. Garnish with chopped parsley, if desired, and serve.
8. Enjoy!

11. Waldorf Salad

Prep Time: 20 Minutes

Cook Time: 20 Minutes

Servings: 4

Ingredients

For the Dressing:

- 6 tablespoons mayonnaise
- 2 tablespoons honey
- 1 tablespoon fresh lemon juice from ½ lemon
- ½ teaspoon salt
- ¼ teaspoon freshly ground black pepper

For the Salad:

- 2 apples chopped or cut into matchsticks
- 1 cup red grapes halved
- 1 cup thinly sliced celery
- 1 cup candied walnuts plus more for garnish
- Mixed greens for serving

Instructions

1. In a medium bowl, whisk the mayonnaise, honey, lemon juice, salt, and pepper together to create the dressing.

2. 6 tablespoons mayonnaise,2 tablespoons honey,1 tablespoon fresh lemon juice,½ teaspoon kosher salt,¼ teaspoon freshly ground black pepper
3. dressing ingredients in a bowl
4. In a large bowl, add the apples, grapes, celery, and candied walnuts. Toss to combine.
5. 2 apples,1 cup red grapes,1 cup thinly sliced celery,1 cup candied walnuts
6. Pour the dressing into the bowl and toss to combine. Plate over greens, top with extra walnuts, and enjoy!
7. Mixed greens.

Prep Time: 5 Minutes

Cook Time: 10 Minutes

Servings: 4

Ingredients

- ½ pound ground beef
- 1 tablespoon taco seasoning store-bought or homemade
- 3 ounces water
- 8 cups chopped lettuce
- 1 cup broken tortilla chips
- ½ cup black beans
- 6 ounces shredded cheddar cheese
- ¾ cup diced tomatoes
- 4 ounces sour cream
- 4 ounces guacamole store-bought or homemade
- ½ cup salsa store-bought or homemade

Instructions

1. In large skillet set over medium-low heat, brown the meat and break into crumbles. Drain any excess grease. Add the meat back into the pan with taco seasoning and water. Cook for 3-5 minutes, or until the sauce has thickened. Remove from heat.
2. ½ pound ground beef,1 tablespoon taco seasoning,3 ounces water

3. cooking ground beef in a skillet
4. While meat is cooking, prepare the lettuce and place it in a large bowl. Once the meat is done, layer it, along with the chips, beans, cheese, tomatoes, sour cream, and guacamole. Serve with salsa or taco sauce.
5. 8 cups chopped lettuce,1 cup broken tortilla chips,½ cup black beans,6 ounces shredded cheddar cheese,¾ cup diced tomatoes,4 ounces sour cream,4 ounces guacamole,½ cup salsa

Prep Time: 30 Minutes

Cook Time: 30 Minutes

Servings: 8

Ingredients

For the Salad:

- ½ head iceberg lettuce chopped
- ½ heart romaine lettuce chopped
- 3 carrots peeled and sliced
- 2 stalks celery sliced
- ¼ red onions thinly sliced
- ½ pint cherry tomatoes halved
- 3 hard-boiled eggs peeled and chopped
- 8 slices bacon cooked crisp and crumbled
- 1 cup croutons
- ½ cup crumbled Feta cheese
- Salt and freshly ground black pepper to taste

For the Dressing:

- ⅓ cup champagne vinegar
- 2 teaspoons freshly squeezed orange juice
- ½ teaspoon freshly grated orange zest from about ¼ orange
- ¼ cup granulated sugar
- 1 tablespoon honey dijon mustard Inglehoffer recommended
- ½ teaspoon fine sea salt
- ½ teaspoon freshly ground black pepper

- 1 teaspoon toasted onion flakes
- ¼ teaspoon crushed red pepper flakes
- 1 cup extra virgin olive oil

Equipment

- High Powered Blender

Instructions

For the Salad

1. Toss all salad ingredients together in a large salad bowl.
2. ½ head iceberg lettuce,½ heart romaine lettuce,3 carrots,2 stalks celery,¼ red onion,½ pint cherry tomatoes,3 hard-boiled eggs,8 slices bacon,1 cup croutons,½ cup crumbled Feta cheese
3. Season with salt and black pepper to taste.
4. Kosher salt and freshly ground black pepper

For the Dressing

1. In the bowl of a blender, add all ingredients except the olive oil. Blend until smooth.
2. ⅓ cup champagne vinegar,½ teaspoon freshly grated orange zest,¼ cup granulated sugar,1 tablespoon honey dijon mustard,½ teaspoon fine sea salt,½ teaspoon freshly ground black pepper,1 teaspoon toasted onion flakes,¼ teaspoon crushed red pepper flakes,2 teaspoons freshly squeezed orange juice
3. Slowly drizzle in the olive oil with the blender on low. Blend on low speed until homogenized, about 1 minute.
4. 1 cup extra virgin olive oil

5. Pour the dressing over the prepared salad and toss to coat.

Prep Time: 10 Minutes

Cook Time: 10 Minutes

Servings: 4

Ingredients

- 2 pounds boneless, skinless chicken breasts
- ¼ cup olive oil
- 4 cloves garlic minced
- ⅓ cup red wine vinegar
- ½ cup finely chopped fresh herbs like parsley, rosemary, thyme, and basil
- ½ teaspoon kosher salt
- ⅛ teaspoon freshly ground black pepper
- Equipment
- Grill or Indoor Grill Pan
- Instant Read Meat Thermometer

Instructions

1. Check the thickness of your chicken breasts. If needed, slice the chicken breasts in half to create thinner pieces, or place the breasts between parchment paper or plastic wrap and pound them to an even thinness.
2. 2 pounds boneless, skinless chicken breasts

3. Whisk the oil, garlic, vinegar, herbs, salt, and pepper together, and pour into a sealable plastic bag or large dish.
4. ¼ cup olive oil,4 cloves garlic,⅓ cup red wine vinegar,½ cup finely chopped fresh herbs,½ teaspoon kosher salt,⅛ teaspoon freshly ground black pepper
5. Add the chicken to the plastic bag or dish and marinate for 2-8 hours.
6. marinating chicken breast in a resealable plastic bag
7. Preheat the grill to medium-high heat (450-500°F).
8. Place the chicken on the grill and cook for around 10 minutes total, flipping the chicken halfway through.
9. Ensure the chicken has reached an internal temperature of 165°F before serving.

Prep Time: 10 Minutes

Cook Time: 7hrs 10 Minutes

Servings: 4

Ingredients

- 1 1/2 pounds shredded rotisserie chicken fully cooked
- 4 cups low sodium chicken broth
- 2 cups water
- 3 cloves garlic minced
- 1 yellow onion diced
- 3 carrots peeled and diced
- 3 stalks celery diced
- 2 15-ounce cans Great Northern beans, drained and rinsed
- 2 bay leaves
- 4 cups baby spinach
- Salt and pepper to taste

Equipment

- Crockpot

Instructions

1. Place chicken, garlic, onion, carrots, celery, beans, and bay leaves into a large slow cooker. Season with salt and pepper to taste.
2. 1 1/2 pounds shredded rotisserie chicken,3 cloves garlic,1 yellow onion,3 carrots,3 stalks celery,2 15-

ounce cans Great Northern beans, drained and rinsed,2 bay leaves,salt and pepper to taste
3. crockpot filled with tuscan chicken soup ingredients
4. Stir in chicken broth and 2 cups water. Stir in spinach. Stir until well combined.
5. 4 cups low sodium chicken broth,2 cups water,4 cups baby spinach
6. slow cooker filled with tuscan soup ingredients
7. Cover and cook on low heat for 7-8 hours or high heat for 3-4 hours.
8. close up on tuscan soup in a crockpot
9. Serve immediately.

Prep Time: 15 Minutes

Cook Time: 15 Minutes

Servings: 6

Ingredients

For the Lemon Vinaigrette:

- 1 lemon juiced (about 3 tablespoons)
- 1 tablespoon minced shallot
- 1 clove garlic grated
- 1 tablespoon Dijon mustard
- 1 teaspoon minced fresh thyme
- ⅓ cup olive oil

For the Orzo Salad:

- 8 ounces dry orzo pasta ½ box
- 1 cup cherry tomatoes halved
- 1 cup Kalamata olives pitted and halved
- 2 ounces feta cheese crumbled
- ¼ cup pine nuts toasted
- Fresh basil, parsley, thyme, or oregano for garnish

Instructions

For the Lemon Vinaigrette

1. Place the lemon juice, shallot, and garlic in a medium bowl and allow it to sit for 5 minutes.
2. 1 lemon,1 tablespoon minced shallot,1 clove garlic

3. overhead view of lemon juice shallot and garlic in a white bowl.
4. Whisk in the Dijon and thyme.
5. 1 tablespoon Dijon mustard,1 teaspoon minced fresh thyme
6. Slowly add the olive oil, whisking constantly until the dressing is fully emulsified. Set aside.
7. ⅓ cup olive oil
8. overhead view of lemon vinaigrette for mediterranean orzo salad in a white bowl.

For the Orzo Salad:

1. Bring a large pot of salted water to a boil. Add the orzo and cook until al dente. Drain the orzo and transfer it to a large bowl.
2. 8 ounces dry orzo pasta
3. Pour the lemon vinaigrette into the bowl with orzo and toss to combine. Set aside to cool slightly (to prevent the feta from melting).
4. overhead view of cooked orzo in a white bowl.
5. When the orzo is cool to the touch, add the tomatoes, olives, feta, and pine nuts. Toss to combine. Garnish with fresh herbs and enjoy.
6. 1 cup cherry tomatoes,1 cup Kalamata olives,2 ounces feta cheese,¼ cup pine nuts,Fresh basil, parsley, thyme, or oregano

Prep Time: 20 Minutes

Cook Time: 10 Minutes

Servings: 6

Ingredients

For the Chimichurri:

- ½ cup packed fresh flat-leaf parsley leaves
- ½ cup packed cilantro leaves
- 2 garlic cloves
- 1 red chili pepper optional
- 2 tablespoons fresh oregano leaves
- ⅓ cup olive oil
- 2 tablespoons red wine vinegar
- ½ teaspoon salt
- ⅛ teaspoon ground black pepper

For the Potatoes:

- 3 tablespoons avocado oil
- ¾ teaspoon salt
- ½ teaspoon ground black pepper
- 4 large russet potatoes each cut into 8 wedges

Instructions

For the Chimichurri

1. Place the parsley, cilantro, garlic, red chili pepper, and oregano in a food processor and pulse until finely chopped.
2. ½ cup packed fresh flat-leaf parsley leaves,½ cup packed cilantro leaves,2 garlic cloves,1 red chili pepper,2 tablespoons fresh oregano leaves
3. overhead view of processed herbs for grilled potato wedges with chimichurri in a food processor.
4. Stir in the olive oil, red wine vinegar, salt, and pepper. Stir well and refrigerate in a lidded container until ready to serve.
5. ⅓ cup olive oil,2 tablespoons red wine vinegar,½ teaspoon kosher salt,⅛ teaspoon ground black pepper
6. oil added to processed herbs for grilled potato wedges with chimichurri in a white bowl.

For the Potatoes

1. Preheat grill to medium (about 400-425°F). Brush grill grates with oil if needed.
2. Place the oil, salt, and pepper in a large bowl with the potato wedges. Toss to coat.
3. 3 tablespoons avocado oil,¾ teaspoon kosher salt,½ teaspoon ground black pepper,4 large russet potatoes
4. potato wedges being oiled in a white bowl.
5. Grill the wedges for 10 minutes, flipping halfway through, until char lines form.
6. Serve the wedges with the chimichurri.

Prep Time: 15 Minutes

Cook Time: 30 Minutes

Servings: 8

Ingredients

- 2 pounds rotisserie chicken shredded
- 3 tablespoons ranch seasoning store-bought or homemade
- 1 head of cauliflower chopped
- 4 cups low-sodium chicken stock
- 2 cups low-sodium chicken broth
- 1 cup water
- 1 pound carrots sliced
- 6 stalks celery sliced
- 1 onion diced
- 1 tablespoon unsalted butter ⅛ stick
- 1 cup Buffalo sauce (store-bought or click for recipe)
- Chopped green onion and blue cheese crumbles optional, for garnish

Equipment

- Immersion Blender

Instructions

1. Boil the cauliflower in a stockpot with the water, ranch seasoning, chicken broth, and chicken stock until very tender; approximately 10 minutes.
2. 3 tablespoons ranch seasoning,1 head of cauliflower,4 cups low-sodium chicken stock,2 cups low-sodium chicken broth,1 cup water
3. soup boiling in a pot
4. While the cauliflower is cooking, sauté the carrots, celery, and onion with the butter. Cook on medium heat until the onions are translucent and the vegetables are fork tender.
5. 1 pound carrots,6 stalks celery,1 onion,1 tablespoon unsalted butter
6. close up on a skillet filled with chopped vegetables
7. Using an immersion blender, blend the cauliflower into a purée in the stockpot. It should blend completely and form a thicker base for the soup. Add the hot sauce and stir.
8. 1 cup Buffalo sauce
9. immersion blender in a pot of soup
10. Add the celery, carrots, and onion to the stockpot and stir.
11. stirring soup in a pot
12. Stir in the chicken pieces and let cook on low for 20-30 minutes
13. 2 pounds rotisserie chicken

Prep Time: 15 Minutes

Cook Time: 30 Minutes

Servings: 4

Ingredients

- ½ cup Balsamic Vinegar
- ½ cup dark brown sugar
- 2 teaspoons olive oil
- 1 (1½-2 pound) salmon fillet bones removed
- 8-12 Campari Tomatoes still on the vine if possible (or Roma tomatoes), halved
- Salt to taste
- Freshly ground black pepper to taste
- 1 teaspoon Italian herb seasoning optional
- 2 tablespoons dark brown sugar
- Fresh basil leaves chopped and whole
- Fresh Mozzarella sliced into ½x½-inch rectangular sticks
- Fresh tomatoes or roma tomatoes cut into ½-inch slices, then each slice cut in half

Equipment

- Baking Sheet
- Instant Read Meat Thermometer

Instructions

1. Preheat oven to 275°F.

2. In a small saucepan, combine the Balsamic Vinegar and brown sugar, bring to a boil, reduce heat to low and simmer until sugar has dissolved and reduction has thickened. Set balsamic reduction aside until ready to use.
3. ½ cup Balsamic Vinegar,½ cup dark brown sugar
4. Brush a baking dish or baking pan (a little larger than length and width of salmon) with 2 teaspoons extra virgin olive oil and place the salmon, skin side down, in the dish. Place the tomatoes, still attached to the vine, on each side of the salmon. Sprinkle the salmon and tomatoes with salt, pepper, favorite herb seasoning, 2 tablespoons brown sugar and the chopped basil.
5. 2 teaspoons olive oil,1 (1½-2 pound) salmon fillet, salt,Freshly ground black pepper,1 teaspoon Italian herb seasoning,2 tablespoons dark brown sugar,Fresh basil leaves,8-12 Campari Tomatoes
6. raw salmon filet on a baking tray with tomatoes on vines
7. With a sharp knife, make three cuts (½-inch deep) along the length of the salmon. One down the middle and one down the middle of each half. The cuts should NOT go all the way through the salmon.
8. cutting slits into salmon to stuff
9. Drizzle the salmon with olive oil then stuff the tomato and mozzarella slices into the cuts of the salmon, alternating between the tomato and mozzarella slices as you go down the salmon.
10. Fresh Mozzarella,Fresh tomatoes or roma tomatoes
11. how to make caprese stuffed salmon
12. Drizzle the salmon with the balsamic-sugar mixture.
13. how to make stuffed salmo with mozzarella and tomatoes

14. Bake the salmon at 275°F for 30 minutes, or until tender when a fork is inserted in the thickest part (or when a meat thermometer registers 115°F in the thickest part). The salmon may look a little underdone – this happens when baked slowly.
15. Leave the salmon in the oven and turn the temperature to BROIL.
16. Broil 2-3 minutes, or until the salmon begins to get a little color. Watch closely.
17. Check the temperature of the salmon with a meat thermometer. The finished salmon should register 120F-125°F.
18. Remove the salmon from the oven and sprinkle with fresh basil leaves.

Prep Time: 20 Minutes

Cook Time: 5 Minutes

Servings: 4

Ingredients

For the Burrito Bowls:

- 2 cups barbacoa meat
- 1 cup chopped butter lettuce
- ½ cup shredded Monterey jack cheese
- ¼ cup plain Greek yogurt
- Cilantro lime cauliflower rice
- Pico de gallon, red tomatillo salsa, and guacamole for serving

For the Cilantro Lime Cauliflower Rice:

- 10 ounces steamable Cauliflower rice 1 bag
- 2 tablespoons chopped cilantro
- 2 limes juiced
- ½ teaspoon ground black pepper

For the Pico de Gallo:

- 2 roma tomatoes diced
- ¼ white onion diced
- ½ lime cut into wedges
- ½ tablespoon chopped cilantro
- ½ teaspoon kosher salt
- ½ teaspoon ground black pepper
- For the Red Tomatillo Salsa:

- 3 tomatillos
- ¼ white onion chopped
- 3 cloves garlic
- 2 chipotle peppers in adobo
- 2 tablespoons chopped cilantro
- 1 teaspoon ground black pepper
- 1 teaspoon A1 steak sauce
- 1 ½ limes juiced

For the Guacamole:

- 1 avocado sliced
- ¼ white onion diced
- ½ lime cut into wedges
- ½ tablespoon chopped cilantro
- ¼ teaspoon salt
- ¼ teaspoon ground black pepper

Instructions

For the Barbacoa Burrito Bowls

1. Prepare the crockpot barbacoa meat and use 2 cups of it in this recipe.
2. 2 cups barbacoa meat
3. Assemble the burrito bowls: Add ½ cup of cilantro lime cauliflower rice to a bowl. Top with ½ cup barbacoa meat, lettuce, cheese, pico de gallo, and a drizzle of tomatillo salsa. Add a dollop of Greek yogurt and guacamole and enjoy.
4. 1 cup chopped butter lettuce, ½ cup shredded Monterey jack cheese, ¼ cup plain Greek yogurt, Pico de gallo, red tomatillo salsa, and guacamole, Cilantro lime cauliflower rice

5. cauliflower rice in a bowl topped with barbacoa meat

For the Cilantro Lime Cauliflower Rice

1. Cook the cauliflower rice according to package instructions. Transfer the steamed cauliflower rice to a bowl. Stir in cilantro, juice from 2 limes, and pepper.
2. 10 ounces steamable Cauliflower rice,2 tablespoons chopped cilantro,2 limes,½ teaspoon ground black pepper
3. cilantro lime cauliflower rice in a glass bowl with a spoon

For the Pico de Gallo

1. In a small bowl combine the tomatoes, onion, juice from ½ lime, cilantro, salt, and pepper.
2. 2 roma tomatoes,¼ white onion,½ lime,½ tablespoon chopped cilantro,½ teaspoon kosher salt,½ teaspoon ground black pepper
3. pico de gallo in a glass bowl with a spoon

For the Red Tomatillo Salsa

1. Preheat the broiler. Cut the tomatillos in half. Place them face down in an oven-safe baking dish. Place the dish 5" from the broiler. Broil for 7 minutes, flip the tomatillos, and broil for 7 more minutes. Let the tomatillos cool for 5 minutes. Add the tomatillos and all remaining ingredients to a food processor bowl. Pulse for 15 seconds or until smooth.
2. 3 tomatillos,¼ white onion,3 cloves garlic,2 chipotle peppers in adobo,2 tablespoons chopped cilantro,1 teaspoon ground black pepper,1 teaspoon A1 steak sauce,1 ½ limes

For the Guacamole

1. In a small bowl, mix the avocado, onion, juice from ½
    lime, cilantro, salt, and black pepper together. Use a
    fork or muddler to mash the avocado and mix
    ingredients.
2. 1 avocado,¼ white onion,½ lime,½ tablespoon
    chopped cilantro,¼ teaspoon kosher salt,¼ teaspoon
    ground black pepper
3. guacamole in a glass bow

21. Easy Baked Spaghetti

Prep Time: 15 Minutes

Cook Time: 30 Minutes

Servings: 6

Ingredients

- 16 ounces dry spaghetti
- 1 pound ground chuck
- 1 tablespoon olive oil
- 1 tablespoon unsalted butter
- 1 medium yellow onion diced
- 3 garlic cloves minced
- 24 ounces marinara sauce one jar of your favorite
- 2 tablespoons chopped fresh basil divided
- 1 cup shredded mozzarella
- ½ cup grated parmesan cheese divided
- salt and freshly ground black pepper to taste

Instructions

1. Preheat oven to 350°F and spray a 13×9 baking dish with nonstick spray.
2. ingredients for baked spaghetti
3. Cook the spaghetti, per package directions, to al dente and drain.
4. 16 ounces dry spaghetti

5. While the spaghetti cooks, brown the beef in a large skillet set over medium heat. Break the beef up with a wooden spoon as it cooks.
6. 1 pound ground chuck
7. ground beef in a skillet with a wood spoon
8. Drain the beef and wipe out the skillet.
9. In the same skillet, add the oil and butter. Add onions and cook until onion has softened and is translucent, about 4-5 minutes. Add minced garlic and cook an additional 30 seconds.
10. 1 tablespoon olive oil,1 tablespoon unsalted butter,1 medium yellow onion,3 garlic cloves
11. minced garlic and cooked chopped onions in a skillet with a wood spoon
12. Add the beef, marinara sauce, 1 tablespoon chopped basil, and ¼ cup grated parmesan cheese. Stir until well combined and season with kosher salt and freshly ground black pepper.
13. 24 ounces marinara sauce,2 tablespoons chopped fresh basil,½ cup grated parmesan cheese,Kosher salt and freshly ground black pepper
14. parmesan cheese, marinara sauce, and ground beef in a skillet with a wood spoon
15. Add the cooked spaghetti to the skillet with the meat sauce mixture and stir until spaghetti is well coated.
16. cooked spaghetti noodles coated with marinara meat sauce in a skillet with 2 wood spoons
17. Transfer the spaghetti mixture to the prepared baking dish and sprinkle with mozzarella and remaining ¼ cup parmesan cheese.
18. 1 cup shredded mozzarella
19. spaghetti mixture topped with cheese in a casserole pan before baking

20. Bake at 350°F for 20-30 minutes or until cheese has melted and the spaghetti is hot throughout.
21. Garnish with the remaining chopped basil and serve.
22. baked spaghetti in a casserole dish

Prep Time: 15 Minutes

Cook Time: 30 Minutes

Servings: 8

Ingredients

- 1 pound ground chuck
- 1 tablespoon olive oil
- 1 small yellow onion diced
- 1 garlic clove minced
- 26 ounces marinara sauce 1 jar
- 1 large egg lightly beaten
- 2 cups small curd cottage cheese 4% milk fat
- 2 cups shredded mozzarella cheese divided
- ¾ cup grated Parmesan cheese divided
- 20 jumbo pasta shells cooked to al dente, per package directions
- Chopped fresh basil leaves for garnish

Instructions

1. Preheat oven to 350°F and spray a 9×13 inch (3 qt.) baking dish with nonstick spray; set aside.
2. Bring a pot of water on the stovetop to a boil. Cook the pasta shells to al dente. After cooking the pasta shells, drain and place them upside down on a baking sheet to dry.
3. 20 jumbo pasta shells
4. cooked pasta shells on a baking sheet

5. In a large skillet, brown the beef on medium heat until cooked through and no pink remains. Drain off the rendered fat.
6. 1 pound ground chuck
7. ground beef in a skillet with a hand holding a wooden spoon
8. Reduce heat to medium-low. In the same skillet with the beef, heat the olive oil and add the onion. Cook until translucent, about 3 minutes. Add the garlic and cook 30 seconds more.
9. 1 tablespoon olive oil,1 small yellow onion,1 garlic clove
10. ground beef, onion, and garlic cooking in a skillet with a hand holding a wooden spoon
11. Reduce heat to low and add the marinara sauce. Simmer uncovered for 30 minutes, stirring occasionally.
12. 26 ounces marinara sauce
13. pouring marinara sauce into saucepan with ground beef, onions, and garlic
14. In a medium bowl, mix the egg, cottage cheese, 1 cup of mozzarella cheese, and ½ cup of parmesan cheese together.
15. 1 large egg,2 cups small curd cottage cheese,2 cups shredded mozzarella cheese,¾ cup grated Parmesan cheese
16. hands mixing cheese filling in a glass bowl for stuffed shells
17. Pour about three quarters of the meat sauce in the bottom of the prepared baking dish.
18. meat marinara sauce in the bottom of a baking dish
19. Stuff the shells with 1 rounded tablespoon of cheese mixture and arrange them on top of the meat sauce,

open-side up. Spoon the remaining meat sauce in-between the shells but not directly on top of the shells.

20. pasta shells stuffed with cheese filling on top of marinara sauce in a baking dish
21. Cover with aluminum foil and bake for 30 minutes. Remove the foil and sprinkle the remaining mozzarella and parmesan cheeses over the shells. Bake 5-7 minutes longer, or until the cheese is melted.
22. hands covering baking dish with aluminum foil
23. Garnish with fresh basil and serve!
24. Chopped fresh basil leaves for garnish
25. hand scooping a baked stuffed pasta shell out of baking pan.

Prep Time: 20 Minutes

Cook Time: 30 Minutes

Servings: 8

Ingredients

For the Soup:

- 2 tablespoon vegetable oil
- 1 medium yellow onion diced
- 4 cloves garlic minced
- 2 jalapenos diced
- 6 cups low-sodium chicken stock
- 2 14.5 ounce fires roasted diced tomatoes w/green chilies
- 1 11 ounce can corn
- 1 14.5 ounce can black beans, rinsed & drained
- 1 tablespoon chili powder
- 2 teaspoon ground cumin
- 1 teaspoon smoked paprika
- 1/8 teaspoon crushed red pepper red pepper flakes, optional
- 3 tablespoons crushed corn tortilla chips
- 3 chicken breasts or 3 cups cubed rotisserie chicken meat
- 2 limes; 1 juiced and 1 cut into wedges for serving
- 1 cup heavy cream
- sea salt to taste
- freshly ground black pepper to taste

For Serving:

- Favorite shredded Mexican cheese
- Corn tortilla chips or strips
- Sour cream
- Fresh cilantro chopped
- Fresh avocado slices
- Lime wedges
- Jalapeno slices

Instructions

For the Soup:

1. Crush enough tortilla chips to make 3 tablespoons and set aside.
2. Heat a Dutch oven over medium heat, and add the vegetable oil.
3. Add onions and cook 3 minutes or until softened and translucent.
4. Add jalapenos and cook an additional 1-minute.
5. Add garlic and cook 30 seconds.
6. Pour in the chicken broth, tomatoes, corn, beans, chili powder, cumin, smoked paprika, crushed red pepper and crushed corn tortilla chips.
7. If using chicken breasts, add them now and reduce the heat to low.
8. Simmer for 20 minutes or until chicken is cooked through.
9. Remove chicken breasts and use two forks to shred. Transfer the shredded chicken back into the pot. (If using chopped rotisserie chicken, add it now.)
10. Add lime juice and heavy cream. Stir well and season with salt & pepper. Cook until heated through.

To Serve:

1. Ladle soup into serving bowls and sprinkle with shredded cheese, corn tortilla chips, a dollop of sour cream and chopped fresh cilantro.
2. Serve a wedge of lime and a few slices of avocado.
3. Enjoy!

Prep Time: 10 Minutes

Cook Time: 20 Minutes

Servings: 4

Ingredients

- 4 boneless skinless chicken breasts
- 1½ cups Ranch dressing
- ½ cup sour cream
- 1-1½ cup grated Parmesan cheese divided
- Salt
- Freshly grated black pepper
- 1/4 cup cooked bacon crumbles
- Garnish: diced fresh parsley

Instructions

1. Heat oven to 375°F and spray an 8 x 11-inch baking dish with cooking spray.
2. If the breasts are uneven in thickness, pound them to an even 1" thickness using a meat pounder.
3. Sprinkle both sides of meat with half the grated Parmesan cheese, salt and freshly ground black pepper. Place the chicken in the prepared baking dish.
4. In a medium bowl, whisk together Ranch dressing and sour cream. Pour the mixture over the chicken breasts and sprinkle with remaining Parmesan cheese.
5. Bake at 375°F for 20-30 minutes or until a meat thermometer inserted in the thickest part of the breast reads 150°F.

6. Set oven to broil and broil the breast an additional 2-4 minutes or until the chicken turns golden. It will burn quickly so watch closely.
7. The chicken is cooked through when the thermometer reads 160°F when inserted in the thickest part of the middle breast.
8. Remove from the oven and sprinkle with cooked bacon crumbles. Allow the chicken to rest a few minutes before serving.
9. Garnish with diced parsley, if desired.
10. Enjoy!

Prep Time: 20 Minutes

Cook Time: 30 Minutes

Servings: 6

Ingredients

- 1 package Delallo Gnocchi Kit
- 1 tablespoon Delallo Extra Virgin Olive Oil
- 2 cloves minced garlic
- 28 ounces Delallo San Marzano crushed tomatoes
- ½ teaspoon salt
- ½ teaspoon black pepper
- 1 teaspoon Italian Seasoning
- 1/2 cup grated parmesan
- 1 1/2 cup shredded mozzarella cheese
- 6 slices whole milk mozzarella cheese
- 12 pepperoni
- Fresh basil for garnish

Instructions

1. Prepare gnocchi according to package instructions. Here is a good post with tips and tricks.
2. Preheat oven to 350F.
3. Heat a large skillet over medium heat. Add the olive oil and allow to heat until glistening.
4. Add the garlic and cook for 1-2 minutes or until fragrant. Add the crushed tomatoes, salt, pepper, and Italian seasoning. Stir to combine. Heat until bubbling/simmering.

5. Reduce heat to low and stir in the grated parmesan and the cooked gnocchi, stirring to combine.
6. Sprinkle with the shredded mozzarella and then layer on the pepperoni and sliced whole milk mozzarella.
7. Bake for 25-30 minutes or until cheese is melted and bubbly.
8. Garnish with fresh basil. Serve and enjoy!

Prep Time: 25 Minutes

Cook Time: 40 Minutes

Servings: 4

Ingredients

- 2 boneless, skinless chicken breasts
- 3 cups buttermilk
- 1 cup all-purpose flour
- 1 tablespoon ground paprika
- 1 tablespoon all-purpose seasoning click link for example
- 1 teaspoon salt
- 1 teaspoon ground black pepper
- 4 tablespoons unsalted butter melted (½ stick)
- ¼ cup fresh flat leaf parsley optional

Instructions

1. CUT chicken breasts in half, lengthwise, to create 4 even portions.
2. 2 boneless, skinless chicken breasts
3. PLACE chicken in a large bowl and marinate in milk for about 20 minutes.
4. 3 cups buttermilk
5. raw chicken breast soaking in buttermilk
6. MIX together flour, paprika, all-purpose spice, salt, and pepper in a medium sized bowl. Set aside.

7. 1 cup all-purpose flour,1 tablespoon ground paprika,1 tablespoon all-purpose seasoning,1 teaspoon kosher salt,1 teaspoon ground black pepper
8. seasoned breading mixture for fried chicken
9. PREHEAT oven to 400°F.
10. Place parchment paper on a 9×13 baking sheet. MELT butter and pour onto the parchment, coating the bottom of the pan/parchment.
11. 4 tablespoons unsalted butter
12. baking tray lined with paper, covered in melted butter
13. Lightly pat each chicken breast with a paper towel to remove excess milk before dipping. DIP each chicken breast, one at a time, in the flour mixture. COAT both sides liberally. PLACE in pan.
14. chicken breast in a bowl, being breaded for fried chicken
15. REPEAT with all four chicken breasts, making sure there is a small amount of room between each breast in the pan. This will allow them to crisp while baking.
16. four pieces of chicken breast covered in flour and breading mixture
17. BAKE at 400°F for 35-40 minutes (or until the breading is golden brown and the juices run clear), flipping each breast after 20 minutes.
18. Remove from oven and transfer to a serving dish. Garnish with parsley if desired. Enjoy!
19. ¼ cup fresh flat leaf parsley.

Prep Time: 15 Minutes

Cook Time: 20 Minutes

Servings: 4

Ingredients

- 4 tilapia filets about 4 oz each
- 3/4 cup grated Parmesan cheese
- 1/8 teaspoon salt see note
- 1 tablespoon lemon pepper
- 1 tablespoon chopped parsley
- 1 tablespoon olive oil
- 1/4 cup shredded Parmesan

For Garnish:

- 1/4 cup diced green onions optional
- Lemon cut into wedges

Instructions

1. Preheat the oven to 400F.
2. Mix together the grated Parmesan, lemon pepper, parsley and salt. Drizzle the tilapia with olive oil, then coat with the cheese mixture, pressing it in lightly with your fingers to make sure it sticks. sprinkle lightly with shredded parmesan. Transfer to foil lined baking sheet.
3. Bake until the fish is opaque in the thickest part, about 10 minutes.

4. To brown further, broil for about 5 more minutes until cheese crust is slightly crispy (watch carefully to make sure fish doesn't burn)
5. Top with green onions and serve and serve with lemon wedges, optional.
6. Enjoy!

Prep Time: 15 Minutes

Cook Time: 2hrs 20 Minutes

Servings: 6

Ingredients

- 1 pound ground beef browned and drained
- 1 onion chopped
- 2 tablespoons chili powder
- 2 teaspoons ground cumin
- ½ teaspoon kosher salt
- 15 ounces kidney beans 1 can, drained
- 10 ounces diced tomatoes with green chilies 1 can, drained
- 6 ounces tomato paste 1 can
- 8 ounces tomato sauce 1 can
- 3 cups low-sodium beef broth
- 2 cups dry elbow macaroni
- 1 cup shredded cheddar cheese
- Chopped fresh cilantro optional, for garnish

Equipment

- Crockpot

Instructions

1. Combine all of the ingredients except the cheese and cilantro in the slow cooker.
2. 1 pound ground beef,1 onion,2 tablespoons chili powder,2 teaspoons ground cumin,½ teaspoon

kosher salt,15 ounces kidney beans,10 ounces diced tomatoes with green chilies,6 ounces tomato paste,8 ounces tomato sauce,3 cups low-sodium beef broth,2 cups dry elbow macaroni

3. Cover and cook on low for 1-2 hours until the pasta is cooked.
4. Sprinkle cheese and fresh cilantro over the top.
5. 1 cup shredded cheddar cheese,Chopped fresh cilantro

29. Crockpot Taco Soup

Prep Time: 20Minutes

Cook Time: 2hrs 20 Minutes

Servings: 8

Ingredients

- ½ tablespoon olive oil
- 1 pound ground beef
- ½ onions chopped
- 2 cups low-sodium beef broth
- 20 ounces diced tomatoes with green chiles 2 cans
- 15 ounces tomato sauce 1 can
- ounces canned black beans 1 can
- 2 cups corn kernels fresh or frozen
- 1 tablespoon chili powder
- 1 teaspoon ground cumin
- 1 teaspoon ground paprika
- ½ teaspoon garlic powder
- ½ teaspoon onion powder
- 1 teaspoon kosher salt
- 1 lime juiced

For Serving (Optional):

- Chopped fresh cilantro
- Shredded cheese
- Tortilla chips
- Equipment
- Crockpot

Instructions

1. Heat the oil in a large skillet set over medium heat.
2. ½ tablespoon olive oil
3. Add in the ground beef and use a wooden spoon to break it up into pieces.
4. 1 pound ground beef
5. Add in the onion. Cook the beef and onion for a few minutes until the meat is browned.
6. ½ onion
7. Transfer the mixture the slow cooker.
8. Add in the beef broth, diced tomatoes with green chiles, tomato sauce, black beans, corn, chili powder, cumin, garlic powder, onion powder, and salt.
9. 2 cups low-sodium beef broth,20 ounces diced tomatoes with green chiles,15 ounces tomato sauce,14.5 ounces canned black beans,2 cups corn kernels,1 tablespoon chili powder,1 teaspoon ground cumin,1 teaspoon ground paprika,½ teaspoon garlic powder,½ teaspoon onion powder,1 teaspoon kosher salt
10. ingredients for crockpot taco soup in a crockpot.
11. Cook on high for 2-4 hours or on low for 4-6 hours.
12. When cooking is complete, give the soup a stir.
13. overhead view of a ladle scooping taco soup from a crockpot.
14. Squeeze in the juice of one lime. Taste, and add more lime juice and/or salt if needed.
15. 1 lime
16. Serve with chopped fresh cilantro, shredded cheese, and tortilla chips.
17. Chopped fresh cilantro,Shredded cheese,Tortilla chips
18. close up of crockpot taco soup in a white bowl.

Prep Time: 10Minutes

Cook Time: 20 Minutes

Servings: 4

Ingredients

- 2 cups low-sodium chicken broth
- 2 cups water
- ½ teaspoon kosher salt
- 1 cup corn grits
- 4 tablespoons unsalted butter ½ stick, cut into 4 pieces
- 1 cup shredded cheddar cheese
- ½ teaspoon ground black pepper
- 6 slices bacon cut into lardons
- 1 pound large shrimp peeled and deveined
- 2 teaspoons Cajun seasoning
- 2 cloves garlic minced
- 2 tablespoons sliced scallion greens plus more for garnish
- Lemon wedges for serving

Equipment

- Cast Iron Skillet

Instructions

1. In a large pot, bring the chicken broth, water, and salt to a boil. Whisk in the grits, reduce the heat to a simmer, and cook, stirring often, until the grits have

absorbed the liquid and are tender, about 10-12 minutes.

2. 2 cups low-sodium chicken broth,2 cups water,½ teaspoon kosher salt,1 cup corn grits
3. how to make cheesy grits
4. Stir in the butter, cheddar, and black pepper. Set aside.
5. 4 tablespoons unsalted butter,1 cup shredded cheddar cheese,½ teaspoon ground black pepper
6. adding grated cheese and pats of butter to a pot of grits
7. In a large cast iron skillet, cook the bacon over medium-high heat until crisp. Turn off the heat, remove with a slotted spoon and set aside. Reserve 2 tablespoons of the bacon grease in the pan and discard the rest.
8. 6 slices bacon
9. Pat the shrimp dry with a paper towel. Toss with the cajun seasoning.
10. 1 pound large shrimp,2 teaspoons Cajun seasoning
11. a bowl of raw shrimp coated in cajun seasoning
12. Return the pan to medium-high heat, add in the shrimp, and garlic. Cook, about 1-2 minutes per side until the shrimp is pink.
13. 2 cloves garlic
14. cooking cajun shrimp in a skillet
15. Remove from the heat, stir in the bacon, scallions, and a squeeze of lemon. Serve over the grits and enjoy!
16. 2 tablespoons sliced scallion greens,Lemon wedges.